Diabetes

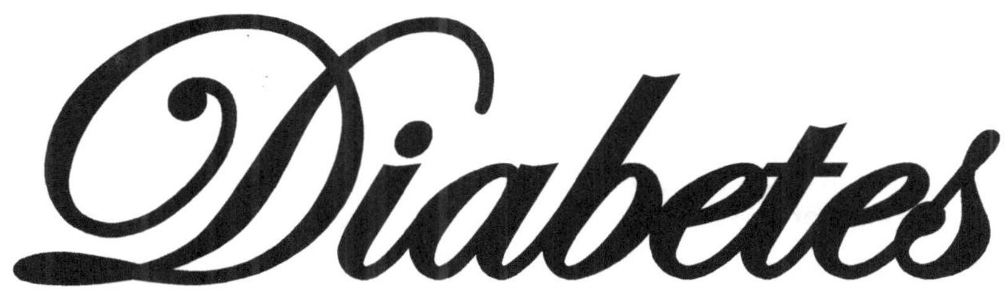

A Guide to Thriving

By

JOEL K. JOHN

TABLE OF CONTENT

Chapter 1: Understanding Diabetes

Types of Diabetes

Type 1 Diabetes:
Type 1 diabetes, also known as juvenile diabetes or insulin-dependent diabetes, is an autoimmune disorder. In this condition, the body's immune system mistakenly attacks and destroys the insulin-producing beta cells in the pancreas. As a result, the pancreas produces little to no insulin. Insulin is crucial for regulating blood sugar levels because it allows glucose to enter the cells to provide energy.
Type 1 diabetes is usually diagnosed in children and young adults, but it can occur at any age. People with Type 1 diabetes must take insulin injections or use insulin pump therapy to manage their blood sugar levels and survive. There is no known cure for Type 1 diabetes, and its exact cause remains unclear, although genetic and

environmental factors are believed to play a role.

Type 2 Diabetes:
Type 2 diabetes is the most common form of diabetes, accounting for the majority of diabetes cases worldwide. In Type 2 diabetes, the body either doesn't produce enough insulin or becomes resistant to the insulin it produces. As a result, glucose builds up in the bloodstream instead of entering the cells, leading to high blood sugar levels.
This type of diabetes is strongly associated with lifestyle factors such as unhealthy diet, lack of physical activity, and obesity. Genetics also plays a role, as Type 2 diabetes tends to run in families. It is more commonly diagnosed in adults, but it can also develop in children and adolescents.

Initially, Type 2 diabetes can often be managed through lifestyle changes, such as adopting a healthy diet, increasing physical activity, and losing weight if necessary.

In some cases, oral medications or insulin therapy may be prescribed to help control blood sugar levels.

Gestational Diabetes:
Gestational diabetes occurs during pregnancy when the body cannot produce enough insulin to meet the increased demands of pregnancy. This condition typically develops around the 24th to 28th week of pregnancy and may resolve after childbirth. However, women who have had gestational diabetes have an increased risk of developing Type 2 diabetes later in life.
Gestational diabetes can be managed through lifestyle changes, such as a balanced diet and regular exercise. In some cases, insulin or oral medications may be necessary to control blood sugar levels during pregnancy.

Other Types:
There are also other rare types of diabetes, such as:

LADA (Latent Autoimmune Diabetes of Adulthood): A slow-progressing form of autoimmune diabetes that shares characteristics with both Type 1 and Type 2 diabetes.

MODY (Maturity-Onset Diabetes of the Young): A genetic form of diabetes that usually starts before age 25 and is caused by a mutation in a specific gene.

Secondary Diabetes: Diabetes that occurs as a result of other medical conditions or certain medications.

It's essential for individuals with diabetes to work closely with healthcare professionals to manage their condition effectively and reduce the risk of complications.

Regular monitoring, proper treatment, and a healthy lifestyle are key to successful diabetes management.

The causes of diabetes can vary depending on the type of diabetes, but in general, genetics and lifestyle factors play a significant role.

Type 1 Diabetes:
The exact cause of Type 1 diabetes is not fully understood, but it is believed to be an autoimmune disorder. In individuals with a genetic predisposition, an environmental trigger, such as a viral infection, may set off an immune response that mistakenly attacks and destroys the insulin-producing beta cells in the pancreas. This destruction leads to a severe deficiency of insulin, and as a result, glucose cannot enter the cells to provide energy, leading to high blood sugar levels.

Genetics: Family history of Type 1 diabetes increases the risk, but not everyone with a family history will develop the condition. Certain genes, such as HLA genes, are associated with an increased susceptibility to Type 1 diabetes.

Environmental Factors: Certain viral infections, especially during childhood, have been linked to an increased risk of developing Type 1 diabetes.

Type 2 Diabetes:
Type 2 diabetes is a complex condition influenced by both genetic and lifestyle factors.
Genetics: Having a family history of Type 2 diabetes increases the risk, but genetics alone does not cause the disease. Multiple genes are associated with Type 2 diabetes, and their interplay with environmental factors determines an individual's risk.

Lifestyle Factors: Unhealthy lifestyle choices significantly contribute to the development of Type 2 diabetes. Factors such as a sedentary lifestyle, poor diet (high in refined carbohydrates, sugary foods, and unhealthy fats), obesity, and insulin resistance (the body's reduced sensitivity to insulin) play a crucial role in the development of Type 2 diabetes.

Gestational Diabetes:
The exact cause of gestational diabetes is not entirely understood, but hormonal changes during pregnancy play a key role.
Hormonal Changes: During pregnancy, the placenta produces hormones that can interfere with the action of insulin, leading to insulin resistance. If the pancreas cannot produce enough insulin to compensate for this resistance, gestational diabetes can develop.

Risk Factors for Type 2 Diabetes and Gestational Diabetes:
Several factors increase the risk of developing Type 2 diabetes and gestational diabetes:

Family History: Having a family history of diabetes increases the risk for both types.

Age: The risk of Type 2 diabetes increases with age, especially after the age of 45.

Obesity: Excess body weight, especially abdominal fat, is a significant risk factor for Type 2 diabetes and gestational diabetes.

Sedentary Lifestyle: Lack of regular physical activity can contribute to insulin resistance and increase the risk of diabetes.

Ethnicity: Certain ethnic groups, such as African Americans, Hispanics, Native Americans, and Asians, have a higher risk of developing Type 2 diabetes.

High Blood Pressure: Hypertension is a risk factor for Type 2 diabetes and gestational diabetes.

Polycystic Ovarian Syndrome (PCOS): Women with PCOS have a higher risk of developing Type 2 diabetes.

Gestational Diabetes History: Women who have had gestational diabetes in a previous pregnancy are at an increased risk of developing Type 2 diabetes later in life.

It's essential to recognize these risk factors and make lifestyle changes to prevent or effectively manage diabetes. Additionally, regular check-ups and screenings are crucial for early detection and proper management of the condition.

How Insulin Works and Its Role in Diabetes

Insulin is a hormone produced by beta cells in the pancreas, and it plays a crucial role in regulating blood sugar levels in the body. Its primary function is to facilitate the uptake of glucose (sugar) from the bloodstream into the cells, where it can be used as a source of energy. Insulin ensures that the cells receive the glucose they need to function properly.

How Insulin Works:
When you eat food, especially carbohydrates, the body breaks down the carbohydrates into glucose, which enters the bloodstream. The rise in blood glucose levels after a meal signals the pancreas to release insulin. Insulin acts as a key that unlocks the cells, allowing glucose to enter.

Insulin binds to specific receptors on the surface of the cell, triggering a series of chemical reactions within the cell. This, in turn, leads to the translocation of glucose transporters (GLUT4) from inside the cell to the cell surface. These transporters facilitate the transport of glucose from the bloodstream into the cell.

Once inside the cell, glucose can be used for energy production or stored as glycogen (a storage form of glucose) in the liver and muscles. This process helps to lower blood glucose levels and maintain them within a healthy range.

Insulin's Role in Diabetes:
In diabetes, there is a problem with insulin production or the way insulin is used in the body, leading to abnormal blood sugar levels. The two main types of diabetes, Type 1 and Type 2, have different underlying mechanisms:

Type 1 Diabetes:
In Type 1 diabetes, the immune system mistakenly attacks and destroys the insulin-producing beta cells in the pancreas. As a result, the pancreas produces little to no insulin. Without sufficient insulin, glucose cannot enter the cells, causing it to accumulate in the

bloodstream. This leads to high blood sugar levels, which can have serious consequences if left uncontrolled.

People with Type 1 diabetes must take insulin injections or use insulin pump therapy to supply their bodies with the insulin they need to regulate blood sugar levels. This is essential for the proper functioning of cells and preventing complications associated with high blood sugar.

Type 2 Diabetes:
In Type 2 diabetes, the body either does not produce enough insulin or becomes resistant to the insulin it produces. Initially, the pancreas may try to compensate for insulin resistance by producing more insulin. However, over time, the pancreas may not be able to keep up with the increased demand for insulin, leading to relative insulin deficiency.

As a result of insulin resistance and/or inadequate insulin production, glucose cannot efficiently enter the cells, and blood sugar levels remain elevated.

Lifestyle factors, such as unhealthy diet, lack of physical activity, and obesity, can contribute to the development of insulin resistance in Type 2 diabetes. Management of Type 2 diabetes may involve lifestyle changes, oral medications, and sometimes insulin therapy to help the body use insulin more effectively or supplement the insulin that the body does not produce.

Insulin is a vital hormone responsible for regulating blood sugar levels by facilitating the uptake of glucose into cells. In diabetes, either the production or the action of insulin is impaired, leading to abnormal blood sugar levels. Effective management of diabetes often involves the administration of insulin or other medications to help maintain proper blood sugar control and prevent complications associated with diabetes.

Chapter 2: Diagnosing Diabetes

Recognizing Common Symptoms of Diabetes

Diabetes can present with a variety of symptoms, and the signs may differ depending on the type of diabetes and the individual's overall health. It's important to be aware of these common symptoms to seek prompt medical attention and get a proper diagnosis. Here are some of the typical symptoms associated with diabetes:

Frequent Urination (Polyuria):
One of the hallmark symptoms of diabetes is frequent urination. When blood sugar levels are high, the kidneys work to remove the excess sugar from the bloodstream by filtering it into the urine. This leads to increased urine production, causing more frequent trips to the bathroom, especially at night (nocturia).

Excessive Thirst (Polydipsia):
The increased urine production caused by high blood sugar levels can result in dehydration, leading to an intense feeling of thirst. Individuals with diabetes often find themselves drinking more water or other fluids to quench their thirst.

Unexplained Weight Loss:
In Type 1 diabetes, where the body lacks insulin, glucose cannot enter the cells for energy. As a result, the body starts breaking down fat and muscle tissues to provide energy, leading to unexplained weight loss despite increased appetite.

Increased Hunger (Polyphagia):
Type 2 diabetes, especially when insulin resistance is present, can lead to hunger even after eating. This happens because the cells are not receiving enough glucose, so the body signals for more food to try to obtain additional energy.

Fatigue and Weakness:
Insufficient glucose getting into the cells can leave individuals feeling tired, fatigued, and weak, as the body's cells are not receiving enough energy.

Blurred Vision:
High blood sugar levels can cause changes in the shape of the lens of the eye, leading to temporary blurring of vision. This symptom may resolve once blood sugar levels are under control.

Slow Healing of Wounds:
High blood sugar can impair the body's ability to heal and fight infections. Cuts and wounds may take longer to heal, and individuals with diabetes may be more susceptible to infections.

Tingling or Numbness:
Uncontrolled diabetes can damage the nerves, leading to a condition called diabetic neuropathy. Symptoms include tingling, numbness, or pain in the hands, feet, or legs.

It's important to note that some people with diabetes, especially in the early stages, may not experience any symptoms or may have very mild symptoms that go unnoticed. This is particularly true for Type 2 diabetes, which can develop gradually over time. Regular check-ups, especially for individuals with risk factors, are crucial for early detection and timely management of diabetes.

If you or someone you know experiences any of these symptoms, especially if there are risk factors for diabetes, it's essential to consult a healthcare professional for proper evaluation and diagnosis. Early diagnosis and effective management are key to preventing complications and maintaining overall health for individuals with diabetes.

Diagnostic Tests and Procedures for Diabetes

Diabetes is diagnosed and monitored through various tests and procedures that measure blood sugar levels and assess how the body processes glucose. These tests help healthcare professionals determine the type of diabetes and establish appropriate management plans. Here are some of the common diagnostic tests and procedures for diabetes:

Fasting Plasma Glucose (FPG) Test: The fasting plasma glucose test is one of the most common tests used to diagnose diabetes. It measures blood glucose levels after an overnight fast (typically 8 hours). A blood sample is taken in the morning before the individual has eaten anything. If the fasting blood sugar level is 126 milligrams per deciliter (mg/dL) or higher on two separate occasions, diabetes is diagnosed.

Oral Glucose Tolerance Test (OGTT):
The oral glucose tolerance test is another
method used to diagnose diabetes,
particularly gestational diabetes. It
involves fasting overnight, then drinking a
sugary solution containing a measured
amount of glucose. Blood samples are
taken at specific intervals (usually 1 and 2
hours after drinking the solution) to
measure how the body responds to the
glucose. A blood sugar level of 200 mg/dL
or higher after 2 hours indicates diabetes.

Hemoglobin A1c (HbA1c) Test:
The HbA1c test provides an average of
blood sugar levels over the past 2 to 3
months. It measures the percentage of
hemoglobin (a protein in red blood cells)
that is coated with sugar. A higher HbA1c
level indicates poorer blood sugar control
over time. An HbA1c level of 6.5% or
higher is indicative of diabetes.

Random Plasma Glucose Test:
In some cases, a random plasma glucose test may be performed, especially if symptoms of diabetes are present. It involves taking a blood sample at any time of the day, regardless of when the person last ate. A blood sugar level of 200 mg/dL or higher, along with symptoms of diabetes, can lead to a diagnosis.

Glycated Albumin (GA) Test:
The glycated albumin test is similar to the HbA1c test but provides a shorter-term average of blood sugar levels over the past few weeks. It is sometimes used in situations where the HbA1c test may not be accurate, such as in individuals with certain types of anemia or hemoglobinopathies.

C-peptide Test:
The C-peptide test measures the level of C-peptide, a byproduct of insulin production, in the blood. This test can help differentiate between Type 1 and Type 2 diabetes.

People with Type 1 diabetes typically have low or undetectable C-peptide levels, while those with Type 2 diabetes usually have normal or elevated C-peptide levels.

These diagnostic tests and procedures, along with a thorough medical history and physical examination, help healthcare professionals determine the presence of diabetes, its type, and the appropriate management plan. Regular monitoring of blood sugar levels and other relevant tests are crucial for assessing diabetes control and preventing complications associated with the condition. It's important for individuals with risk factors for diabetes or those experiencing symptoms to seek medical attention promptly for proper evaluation and diagnosis.

Type 1 and Type 2 diabetes are two distinct forms of diabetes, each with its own underlying causes, age of onset, and treatment approaches. It's important to differentiate between the two types to provide appropriate management and care. Here are the key factors that help distinguish Type 1 and Type 2 diabetes:

Underlying Causes:
Type 1 Diabetes: Type 1 diabetes is an autoimmune condition. It occurs when the body's immune system mistakenly attacks and destroys the insulin-producing beta cells in the pancreas. As a result, the pancreas produces little to no insulin, leading to an absolute insulin deficiency. The exact cause of this autoimmune reaction is not fully understood, but genetic and environmental factors are believed to play a role.

Type 2 Diabetes: Type 2 diabetes is characterized by insulin resistance, where the body's cells do not respond effectively to insulin. Initially, the pancreas may produce extra insulin to compensate for this resistance. However, over time, the pancreas may not be able to maintain sufficient insulin production, leading to a relative insulin deficiency. Type 2 diabetes is strongly associated with lifestyle factors, such as unhealthy diet, lack of physical activity, and obesity. Genetics also plays a role in the development of Type 2 diabetes.

Age of Onset:

Type 1 Diabetes: Type 1 diabetes is often diagnosed in children, adolescents, or young adults, although it can occur at any age. It is sometimes referred to as juvenile diabetes due to its higher incidence in younger age groups.

Type 2 Diabetes: Type 2 diabetes is more commonly diagnosed in adults, particularly in those over the age of 45.

However, due to the rise in childhood obesity and sedentary lifestyles, Type 2 diabetes is increasingly being diagnosed in children and adolescents as well.

Insulin Dependency:
Type 1 Diabetes: People with Type 1 diabetes require insulin therapy to survive because their bodies do not produce enough insulin. Insulin is typically administered through injections or insulin pump therapy.

Type 2 Diabetes: Initially, people with Type 2 diabetes may not require insulin treatment and can manage their condition through lifestyle changes, oral medications, or other non-insulin injectable medications. However, as the disease progresses, some individuals with Type 2 diabetes may eventually require insulin therapy to control their blood sugar levels.

Body Weight:

Type 1 Diabetes: Type 1 diabetes is not associated with body weight. People with Type 1 diabetes may have a normal, underweight, or overweight body composition.

Type 2 Diabetes: Type 2 diabetes is often associated with overweight or obesity. Excess body weight, especially abdominal fat, is a significant risk factor for developing Type 2 diabetes.

Ketosis:

Type 1 Diabetes: Due to the absolute lack of insulin, people with Type 1 diabetes are at risk of developing diabetic ketoacidosis (DKA) if their blood sugar levels become very high. DKA is a life-threatening condition characterized by the buildup of ketones in the blood.

Type 2 Diabetes: Ketosis is not a common feature of Type 2 diabetes. However, if insulin deficiency becomes severe, as in advanced cases or during times of extreme stress or illness, individuals with Type 2 diabetes may also develop ketosis or a condition called hyperosmolar hyperglycemic state (HHS).

It's important to remember that there are other forms of diabetes as well, such as gestational diabetes, LADA (Latent Autoimmune Diabetes of Adulthood), and MODY (Maturity-Onset Diabetes of the Young), each with its unique characteristics and treatment considerations. Accurate diagnosis and proper differentiation between the types of diabetes are crucial for effective management and improved outcomes for individuals living with diabetes. A healthcare professional or endocrinologist can conduct the necessary tests and assessments to make a definitive diagnosis and develop a personalized treatment plan.

Chapter 3: Building a Management Team

The Importance of Healthcare Professionals in Diabetes Care

Diabetes is a complex and chronic condition that requires ongoing management and support to prevent complications and maintain overall health. Healthcare professionals play a critical role in diabetes care by providing education, guidance, monitoring, and personalized treatment plans. Here are some reasons why healthcare professionals are essential for effective diabetes care:

Diagnosis and Treatment: Healthcare professionals, including doctors, endocrinologists, and diabetes educators, are responsible for diagnosing diabetes accurately. They assess the patient's medical history, symptoms, and conduct diagnostic tests to determine the type of diabetes and its severity. Based on the diagnosis, they develop personalized treatment plans, which may include lifestyle modifications, medication, and insulin therapy.

Education and Self-Management: Proper education is vital for individuals with diabetes to understand their condition and learn how to manage it effectively. Healthcare professionals provide comprehensive diabetes education, covering topics such as blood sugar monitoring, medication management, healthy eating, physical activity, and stress management. This empowers patients to take an active role in their self-care and make informed decisions about their health.

Blood Sugar Monitoring and Management: Regular monitoring of blood sugar levels is crucial for diabetes management. Healthcare professionals guide patients on how and when to check their blood sugar levels, interpret the results, and make appropriate adjustments to their treatment plan based on the readings.

Medication Management: Healthcare professionals prescribe and manage diabetes medications, including insulin, oral medications, or other injectable medications. They ensure that patients take the right dosage at the correct times and monitor for any potential side effects or interactions with other medications.

Lifestyle Counseling: Healthcare professionals help patients adopt healthy lifestyle behaviors, such as a balanced diet, regular physical activity, weight management, and smoking cessation. These lifestyle changes can significantly improve blood sugar control and reduce the risk of diabetes-related complications.

Preventing Complications: Early detection and intervention are crucial for preventing or delaying diabetes-related complications.

Healthcare professionals monitor patients for signs of complications, such as nerve damage, kidney problems, eye issues, and heart disease. They implement preventive strategies and refer patients to specialists when needed.

Emotional Support: Managing diabetes can be emotionally challenging, and healthcare professionals offer emotional support and counseling to help patients cope with the emotional aspects of the condition. They address fears, anxiety, and depression that can arise from living with a chronic illness.

Regular Follow-ups: Healthcare professionals schedule regular follow-up appointments to monitor diabetes control, review treatment plans, and make adjustments as needed. These follow-ups are essential for tracking progress, addressing any issues, and maintaining motivation for long-term diabetes management.

Emergency Planning: Healthcare professionals educate patients about managing diabetes during special circumstances, such as illness, travel, or surgery. They provide guidance on how to handle sick days, adjust medications during travel, and maintain good blood sugar control during challenging situations.

Advocacy and Support: Healthcare professionals advocate for diabetes awareness, support, and access to resources. They collaborate with other members of the diabetes management team, including dieticians, nurses, pharmacists, and specialists, to provide comprehensive and coordinated care.

Healthcare professionals are indispensable in diabetes care, offering expertise, support, and guidance to individuals with diabetes. With their help, patients can achieve better blood sugar control, reduce the risk of complications, and lead healthier lives while living with diabetes.

Creating a Personalized Diabetes Management Plan

Managing diabetes effectively requires a personalized approach that considers an individual's unique needs, lifestyle, and medical condition. A personalized diabetes management plan aims to achieve optimal blood sugar control, prevent complications, and improve overall well-being. Here are the key steps involved in creating a personalized diabetes management plan:

Medical Assessment and Education: The first step is to undergo a comprehensive medical assessment by a healthcare professional, such as a doctor or an endocrinologist. This assessment includes a review of the individual's medical history, current symptoms, and any previous diabetes-related complications. The healthcare professional will also conduct necessary diagnostic tests,

such as blood sugar tests (fasting plasma glucose, HbA1c, etc.), lipid profile, kidney function tests, and eye exams.
Education is a crucial component of the management plan. The healthcare team will provide comprehensive diabetes education, covering various aspects of diabetes care, including blood sugar monitoring, medication management, healthy eating, physical activity, and the importance of stress management and emotional support.

Goal Setting:
After the initial assessment and education, the individual and healthcare team work together to set specific and achievable goals for diabetes management. These goals may include target blood sugar levels, weight management targets, dietary goals, and exercise objectives. Setting realistic and personalized goals helps to maintain motivation and track progress effectively.

Blood Sugar Monitoring:
Regular blood sugar monitoring is essential for diabetes management. The healthcare team will guide the individual on how and when to check blood sugar levels. Based on the results, adjustments to diet, medication, or insulin therapy may be made to maintain blood sugar within the target range.

Meal Planning:
A personalized meal plan is designed to meet the individual's nutritional needs while managing blood sugar levels. The dietitian or diabetes educator will help create a balanced meal plan that emphasizes whole grains, fruits, vegetables, lean proteins, and healthy fats. Carbohydrate counting and portion control may also be incorporated into the meal plan to manage post-meal blood sugar spikes effectively.

Physical Activity:
The healthcare team will recommend an exercise routine tailored to the individual's fitness level, preferences, and health condition. Regular physical activity helps improve insulin sensitivity, control blood sugar levels, manage weight, and enhance overall cardiovascular health. The exercise plan may include a combination of aerobic activities, strength training, and flexibility exercises.

Medication and Insulin Therapy:
Depending on the type of diabetes and its progression, medication or insulin therapy may be necessary to achieve optimal blood sugar control. The healthcare team will prescribe and adjust medications as needed, considering the individual's response and potential side effects. For those on insulin therapy, proper administration, storage, and injection techniques will be taught.

Managing Other Health Conditions:
Diabetes often coexists with other health
conditions such as hypertension,
dyslipidemia, and kidney problems. The
personalized management plan should
address these conditions and incorporate
strategies to manage them effectively.

Regular Follow-ups:
Regular follow-up appointments with the
healthcare team are crucial for reviewing
progress, adjusting the management plan
as needed, and addressing any concerns or
challenges. The frequency of follow-ups
may vary based on the individual's
condition and diabetes control.

**Emotional Support and Coping
Strategies**:
Living with diabetes can be emotionally
challenging, and emotional support is
essential for successful management. The
healthcare team provides emotional
support and helps the individual develop
coping strategies to deal with the stress
and emotional aspects of diabetes.

Emergency Preparedness:
The management plan should include guidelines for handling sick days, managing diabetes during travel, and other special circumstances. Emergency contacts and action plans for severe hypoglycemia or hyperglycemia should also be part of the plan.

Creating a personalized diabetes management plan involves a collaborative effort between the individual with diabetes and the healthcare team. With regular monitoring, ongoing support, and adjustments as needed, individuals can lead healthier lives and effectively manage their diabetes to reduce the risk of complications and improve overall quality of life.

Managing diabetes effectively requires a multidisciplinary approach that involves a team of healthcare professionals with specialized expertise in diabetes care. Integrating dietitians, diabetes educators, and specialists into your diabetes care team can significantly improve outcomes and provide comprehensive support. Here's how each member contributes to diabetes management:

Dietitians or Nutritionists:

Dietitians or nutritionists play a central role in diabetes care by providing expert guidance on diet and meal planning. They help individuals with diabetes develop personalized meal plans that promote blood sugar control, manage weight, and address specific dietary needs. Dietitians educate patients about carbohydrate counting, glycemic index, portion control, and the importance of balanced nutrition.

Their contributions include:

-Creating personalized meal plans that align with the individual's preferences, cultural background, and health goals.
-Teaching carbohydrate counting to help manage blood sugar levels.
-Educating about the role of different nutrients and how they impact diabetes management.
-Providing practical tips for making healthier food choices, cooking techniques, and label reading.
-Addressing other nutritional concerns, such as managing cholesterol, blood pressure, and weight.

Diabetes Educators:
Diabetes educators are healthcare professionals specially trained to educate and support individuals living with diabetes. They play a crucial role in empowering patients to take control of their diabetes self-management. Diabetes educators provide ongoing education, guidance, and problem-solving strategies

to help patients overcome barriers and achieve diabetes management goals.

Their contributions include:

-Providing comprehensive diabetes education, covering various aspects of diabetes care, including blood sugar monitoring, medication management, exercise, and stress management.
-Teaching self-injection techniques for insulin and other injectable medications.
-Offering support for incorporating lifestyle changes into daily routines.
-Assisting with setting personalized diabetes management goals and developing action plans to achieve them.
-Addressing psychological and emotional aspects of living with diabetes, including coping with stress, anxiety, and depression.

Diabetes Specialists (Endocrinologists): Diabetes specialists, such as endocrinologists, are medical doctors with expertise in the endocrine system, which includes the pancreas and hormones like insulin. They play a critical role in the diagnosis, treatment, and management of diabetes, especially in cases where more complex care is required.

Their contributions include:

-Making an accurate diagnosis of the type of diabetes and determining the best treatment approach.
-Prescribing and adjusting diabetes medications, including insulin therapy.
-Addressing other endocrine-related issues that may impact diabetes management.
-Managing diabetes-related complications and coordinating care with other specialists as needed.
-Providing guidance on the integration of new technologies and treatment options into diabetes care.

The collaboration between dietitians, diabetes educators, and diabetes specialists creates a holistic and patient-centered approach to diabetes management. By working together as a team, they can address the various aspects of diabetes care comprehensively, optimize blood sugar control, prevent complications, and improve overall quality of life for individuals with diabetes.

Regular communication and coordination among team members ensure that all aspects of the management plan are aligned, and any necessary adjustments are made promptly. This integrated approach not only enhances patient outcomes but also empowers individuals with diabetes to become active participants in their own care, leading to better self-management and long-term success in diabetes management.

Chapter 4: Blood Glucose Monitoring

Understanding Blood Glucose Levels

Blood glucose, also known as blood sugar, refers to the amount of glucose present in the bloodstream at any given time. Glucose is a type of sugar that serves as the primary source of energy for the body's cells. Understanding blood glucose levels is essential for individuals with diabetes, as it plays a crucial role in diabetes management and overall health.

Normal Blood Glucose Levels:
For individuals without diabetes, blood glucose levels are generally well-regulated and maintained within a relatively narrow range throughout the day. Normal blood glucose levels can vary slightly based on factors such as age, time of day, and whether the person has recently eaten. Here are the general guidelines for normal blood glucose levels:

Fasting Blood Glucose (before meals):
70-99 milligrams per deciliter (mg/dL) or
3.9-5.5 millimoles per liter (mmol/L).

**Postprandial Blood Glucose (1-2 hours
after meals)**: Less than 140 mg/dL or less
than 7.8 mmol/L.

**Understanding Blood Glucose Levels in
Diabetes**:
In diabetes, the body's ability to regulate
blood glucose levels is impaired, leading
to either high blood sugar (hyperglycemia)
or low blood sugar (hypoglycemia).
Monitoring blood glucose levels is crucial
for individuals with diabetes to prevent
complications and maintain optimal health.
Here are the key aspects of understanding
blood glucose levels in diabetes:

Hyperglycemia:
Hyperglycemia occurs when blood
glucose levels are consistently higher than
the target range. This can happen due to
various factors, such as inadequate insulin
production (in Type 1 diabetes),

insulin resistance (in Type 2 diabetes), illness, stress, certain medications, or consuming too many carbohydrates. Symptoms of hyperglycemia include frequent urination, excessive thirst, fatigue, blurred vision, and slow wound healing. If left untreated, hyperglycemia can lead to diabetic ketoacidosis (DKA) in Type 1 diabetes or hyperosmolar hyperglycemic state (HHS) in Type 2 diabetes, both of which are serious and potentially life-threatening conditions.

Hypoglycemia:
Hypoglycemia, or low blood sugar, occurs when blood glucose levels drop below the target range. This can happen if a person with diabetes takes too much insulin or diabetes medication, skips or delays meals, or engages in vigorous physical activity without adjusting their treatment plan. Symptoms of hypoglycemia include shakiness, sweating, dizziness, confusion, and rapid heartbeat. If left untreated, severe hypoglycemia can lead to loss of consciousness and requires immediate

treatment with a fast-acting source of glucose, such as glucose tablets or gel.

Blood Glucose Monitoring:
Regular blood glucose monitoring is essential for individuals with diabetes to understand how their body responds to food, exercise, medications, and other factors. Monitoring allows individuals to make informed decisions about their diabetes management, adjust insulin doses, and identify patterns or trends in blood glucose levels.
Blood glucose can be measured using a blood glucose meter, which requires a small drop of blood obtained by pricking the finger with a lancet. Continuous glucose monitoring (CGM) systems are also available, providing real-time glucose readings and trends throughout the day.

Target Blood Glucose Levels:
Individuals with diabetes work with their healthcare team to set target blood glucose levels based on their age, type of diabetes, overall health, and individual goals. The

targets for blood glucose levels may vary before and after meals, during physical activity, and at different times of the day. Maintaining blood glucose levels within the target range reduces the risk of diabetes-related complications and improves overall well-being.

Long-Term Blood Glucose Control: HbA1c (hemoglobin A1c) is a measure of the average blood glucose levels over the past 2 to 3 months. It is used to assess long-term blood glucose control. The American Diabetes Association (ADA) recommends an HbA1c goal of less than 7% for most adults with diabetes. Understanding blood glucose levels is a fundamental aspect of diabetes self-management. It empowers individuals with diabetes to make informed decisions, take appropriate actions to correct high or low blood sugar, and work towards achieving optimal diabetes control and overall health.

Regular communication with healthcare professionals is essential to interpret blood glucose data effectively and make necessary adjustments to the diabetes management plan.

Glucose monitoring devices are essential tools for individuals with diabetes to measure their blood sugar levels and manage their condition effectively. There are several types of glucose monitoring devices available, ranging from traditional fingerstick blood glucose meters to continuous glucose monitoring (CGM) systems. Here's a guide to selecting and using glucose monitoring devices:

Types of Glucose Monitoring Devices:

a. **Blood Glucose Meters**:
Blood glucose meters are portable devices that measure blood sugar levels from a small drop of blood obtained by pricking the finger with a lancet.
They provide real-time readings and are suitable for self-monitoring at home or on-the-go.
Most blood glucose meters display results within seconds.

b. **Continuous Glucose Monitoring (CGM) Systems**:
CGM systems consist of a small sensor inserted under the skin, which measures interstitial glucose levels (glucose in the fluid between cells).
The sensor continuously sends glucose readings to a receiver or a compatible smartphone or smartwatch.
CGM systems provide real-time glucose data, including trend arrows indicating the direction and speed of glucose changes.
Some CGM systems can also provide alerts for high and low glucose levels.

Factors to Consider when Selecting Glucose Monitoring Devices:
a. **Accuracy**: Look for devices with proven accuracy. Check reviews and consult with healthcare professionals to select a reliable glucose monitoring device.

b. **Ease of Use**: Consider the device's user-friendliness, especially if you plan to use it frequently or have difficulty with technology.

c. **Cost**: Compare the cost of the glucose monitoring device and test strips (for blood glucose meters) or sensors (for CGM systems). Some CGM systems may have higher initial costs but can provide more comprehensive glucose data.

d. **Insurance Coverage**: Check if your health insurance covers glucose monitoring devices and supplies. Some insurers may have preferred brands or coverage limitations.

e. **Data Storage and Connectivity**: Consider devices that can store glucose data, connect to smartphones or computers, and sync with diabetes management apps for easy tracking and analysis.

f. **Alarm Features**: For CGM systems, assess the availability of customizable alarms for high and low glucose levels, especially if you need additional support for glucose management.

How to Use Glucose Monitoring Devices:

a. **Blood Glucose Meters**:
-Wash your hands with warm, soapy water, and dry them thoroughly.
-Insert a test strip into the meter.
-Use a lancet device to prick the side of your fingertip gently to obtain a small drop of blood.
-Touch the drop of blood to the test strip on the meter.
-The meter will display your blood glucose reading.

b. **Continuous Glucose Monitoring (CGM) Systems**:
-Follow the manufacturer's instructions for sensor insertion.
-Pair the CGM system's receiver or transmitter with a compatible device (smartphone, smartwatch, or receiver).
-Calibrate the CGM system if required, according to the manufacturer's guidelines.
-Regularly check the glucose readings on the receiver or connected device for real-time data.

Tips for Accurate Glucose Monitoring:
a. Regularly calibrate CGM systems, if necessary, to ensure accurate readings.

b. Keep your glucose monitoring devices and test strips or sensors in a cool, dry place.

c. Clean your blood glucose meter and CGM sensor site regularly to prevent contamination.

d. Replace lancets and CGM sensors according to the manufacturer's recommendations.

e. Compare glucose meter readings with lab-based blood glucose tests periodically to check for accuracy.

f. Be aware that certain factors, such as medications, food intake, stress, and physical activity, can influence blood glucose readings.

Remember that glucose monitoring devices are valuable tools, but they are not a substitute for regular check-ups with healthcare professionals. Discuss your glucose data and diabetes management plan with your healthcare team to make informed decisions and achieve optimal blood sugar control.

Interpreting Blood Glucose Data and Adjusting Treatment

Interpreting blood glucose data is a crucial aspect of diabetes management. Regular monitoring of blood sugar levels helps individuals with diabetes understand how their bodies respond to various factors, such as food, physical activity, medications, and stress. By interpreting the data, individuals and their healthcare team can make informed decisions to adjust the treatment plan and optimize blood sugar control. Here are the key steps in interpreting blood glucose data and making treatment adjustments:

Keep a Blood Glucose Log:
Maintaining a blood glucose log or using diabetes management apps can help track blood sugar readings over time. It provides a clear picture of glucose patterns throughout the day, including fasting, pre-meal, post-meal, and bedtime readings.

The log may also include notes about food intake, exercise, medication dosages, and any factors that might affect blood sugar levels.

Identify Patterns and Trends:
Analyze the blood glucose data to identify patterns and trends. Look for consistent high or low blood sugar readings at specific times of the day or after certain meals. Pay attention to how different factors, such as meals, physical activity, or medication, affect blood sugar levels. Identifying patterns helps pinpoint areas that require adjustment in the treatment plan.

Understand Target Ranges:
Work with your healthcare team to set target blood glucose ranges for different times of the day. These targets may vary depending on individual factors, age, type of diabetes, overall health, and treatment goals.

The American Diabetes Association (ADA) recommends the following general targets:

Fasting blood glucose (before meals): 80-130 mg/dL (4.4-7.2 mmol/L)

Postprandial blood glucose (1-2 hours after meals): Less than 180 mg/dL (10.0 mmol/L)

Adjusting Treatment:
Based on the blood glucose data and identified patterns, the healthcare team may suggest adjustments to the treatment plan. Treatment adjustments may include:

a. **Medication Changes**: For individuals with Type 2 diabetes, adjustments to oral medications or injectable non-insulin medications may be recommended to achieve better blood sugar control. For those with Type 1 diabetes or advanced Type 2 diabetes, insulin dosage may need to be modified.

b. **Insulin Therapy**: If using insulin, the healthcare team may suggest changes in the type of insulin, dosage, or timing of injections to match meal patterns and activity levels.

c. **Meal Planning**: Modifying the content and timing of meals, as well as carbohydrate counting, can help achieve more stable blood sugar levels after eating.

d. **Physical Activity**: Adjusting the intensity, duration, or timing of exercise can impact blood sugar levels. Coordination with the healthcare team ensures safe adjustments to exercise routines.

e. **Stress Management**: Stress can affect blood sugar levels, so implementing stress reduction techniques may be beneficial.

Avoid Overreacting to Individual Readings:
Remember that blood glucose levels can fluctuate throughout the day due to various factors. Avoid making drastic treatment changes based on individual readings. Instead, focus on identifying trends and making gradual adjustments to the treatment plan.

Regular Follow-ups:
Schedule regular follow-up appointments with your healthcare team to review blood glucose data, treatment adjustments, and progress. Regular monitoring and communication with the healthcare team ensure that the diabetes management plan remains effective and tailored to individual needs.

Seek Support and Education:
Engage in diabetes education and support programs to enhance your understanding of diabetes management and blood glucose interpretation.

Diabetes educators, support groups, and online resources can provide valuable insights and motivation.

Interpreting blood glucose data is an ongoing process that requires collaboration between individuals with diabetes and their healthcare team. By analyzing patterns and trends, making appropriate treatment adjustments, and maintaining open communication, individuals can achieve better blood sugar control, reduce the risk of complications, and improve overall well-being while living with diabetes.

Chapter 5: Healthy Eating for Diabetes

The Role of Diet in Diabetes Management

Diet plays a fundamental role in the management of diabetes. What and when you eat directly affect your blood sugar levels, insulin sensitivity, and overall health. A well-balanced and individualized diet can help individuals with diabetes achieve better blood sugar control, manage body weight, reduce the risk of complications, and improve overall well-being. Here are the key aspects of the role of diet in diabetes management:

Balancing Carbohydrates, Protein, and Fat:
Carbohydrates have the most significant impact on blood sugar levels because they break down into glucose during digestion. Managing carbohydrate intake is crucial for blood sugar control.

Focus on consuming complex carbohydrates from whole grains, fruits, vegetables, and legumes, which have a slower impact on blood sugar compared to simple sugars.
Proteins and fats also influence blood sugar levels, but to a lesser extent than carbohydrates. Including lean proteins and healthy fats in meals can help slow down the absorption of carbohydrates and provide sustained energy.

Carbohydrate Counting and Glycemic Index:
Carbohydrate counting is a method of tracking the number of carbohydrates in meals to help manage blood sugar levels. Knowing the carbohydrate content of foods and adjusting portion sizes accordingly can assist in achieving consistent blood sugar control.
The glycemic index (GI) ranks foods based on how quickly they raise blood sugar levels. Foods with a low GI have a slower impact on blood sugar, making them beneficial for people with diabetes.

Incorporating more low-GI foods can contribute to better blood sugar management.

Meal Timing and Frequency:
Spacing meals evenly throughout the day and avoiding prolonged periods without eating can help stabilize blood sugar levels. Eating regular, balanced meals can prevent extreme fluctuations in blood glucose and avoid overeating at subsequent meals.

Portion Control and Caloric Intake:
Maintaining a healthy body weight is essential for managing diabetes. Portion control and managing caloric intake are vital for weight management. Balancing energy intake with energy expenditure helps prevent weight gain or promotes weight loss if needed.

Hydration:
Staying well-hydrated is essential for everyone, including individuals with diabetes.

Drinking water and low-calorie beverages can help maintain proper hydration without causing significant fluctuations in blood sugar.

Individualized Meal Plans:
Diabetes management is not a one-size-fits-all approach. Meal plans should be personalized based on an individual's preferences, cultural background, age, activity level, and type of diabetes. Working with a registered dietitian or diabetes educator can help create a customized meal plan that suits specific needs and goals.

Consistency and Education:
Consistency in eating patterns, meal timing, and carbohydrate distribution can promote stable blood sugar levels. Regular diabetes education helps individuals understand how food choices impact blood sugar and empowers them to make informed decisions about their diet.

Managing Special Occasions and Holidays:
During special occasions or holidays with festive meals, individuals with diabetes can still enjoy the festivities while being mindful of their food choices and portions. Planning ahead and making adjustments as needed can help maintain blood sugar control during these times.

Remember that diet alone cannot replace medication or insulin therapy for diabetes management. However, combining a healthy diet with other aspects of diabetes care, such as physical activity and medication adherence, forms a comprehensive approach to managing diabetes effectively.

As with any significant dietary changes, it's essential to work closely with a healthcare team, including a registered dietitian or diabetes educator, to develop a personalized meal plan that aligns with individual health goals and medical conditions.

By making smart food choices and practicing portion control, individuals with diabetes can enjoy a well-balanced diet that supports optimal blood sugar control and overall well-being.

Carbohydrate Counting and Glycemic Index in Diabetes Management

Carbohydrate counting and glycemic index are two important dietary strategies used in diabetes management. These approaches help individuals with diabetes make informed food choices to manage blood sugar levels effectively. Both techniques focus on understanding how carbohydrates in foods impact blood sugar levels and play a crucial role in meal planning for people with diabetes.

Carbohydrate Counting:
Carbohydrate counting is a method used to track the number of carbohydrates consumed in meals and snacks. Carbohydrates are the primary nutrient that significantly influences blood sugar levels as they are broken down into glucose during digestion. By monitoring and managing carbohydrate intake, individuals with diabetes can better control their blood sugar levels and adjust

their insulin or medication dosages accordingly.

Steps for Carbohydrate Counting:

a. **Identify Carbohydrate Sources**: Learn to recognize foods that contain carbohydrates. Carbohydrates are found in various foods, including grains, fruits, vegetables, legumes, dairy products, and sweets.

b. **Measure Portion Sizes**: Accurately measure or estimate the portion sizes of carbohydrate-containing foods consumed. Pay attention to serving sizes mentioned on food labels.

c. **Calculate Carbohydrate Content**: Use food labels, carbohydrate counting books, or mobile applications to determine the carbohydrate content of each food item. The carbohydrate content is usually measured in grams.

d. **Track Carbohydrate Intake**: Keep a record of the total grams of carbohydrates consumed at each meal and snack throughout the day.

e. **Adjust Insulin or Medication Dosage**: Based on carbohydrate intake and blood sugar readings, individuals can work with their healthcare team to adjust insulin or medication dosages to match their carbohydrate consumption.

Glycemic Index (GI):
The glycemic index (GI) is a ranking system that measures how quickly carbohydrates in foods raise blood sugar levels. It assigns a numerical value to foods based on their effect on blood glucose compared to a reference food (usually glucose or white bread).

Low GI Foods: Foods with a low GI (55 or less) are digested more slowly, resulting in a gradual and more stable increase in blood sugar levels. These foods are considered beneficial for individuals with diabetes as they help prevent rapid spikes in blood sugar.

Medium GI Foods: Foods with a medium GI (56 to 69) cause a moderate increase in blood sugar levels.

High GI Foods: Foods with a high GI (70 or above) are rapidly digested, leading to a quick and sharp increase in blood sugar levels. High GI foods are generally best consumed in moderation by individuals with diabetes.

Using Glycemic Index in Diabetes Management:

a. **Choosing Low GI Foods**: Including more low GI foods in the diet can help stabilize blood sugar levels and promote better glycemic control. Low GI foods include whole grains, most fruits (except watermelon and ripe bananas), non-starchy vegetables, legumes, and dairy products.

b. **Balancing with Other Nutrients**: While GI is a useful tool, it is essential to consider the overall nutritional profile of foods. Combining low GI foods with proteins, healthy fats, and fiber-rich options can further slow down the digestion of carbohydrates and improve overall meal balance.

c. **Individual Variability**: It's important to note that the GI of a food can vary among individuals and when foods are consumed in combination. Additionally, food preparation methods and ripeness can also influence the GI of certain foods.

Integrating carbohydrate counting and glycemic index into diabetes management empowers individuals to make informed food choices and maintain better blood sugar control. These approaches promote flexibility in food selection while allowing for individual preferences and cultural practices.

Working with a registered dietitian or diabetes educator can further enhance the application of these techniques, ensuring personalized and effective dietary strategies for individuals with diabetes.

Meal Planning and Portion Control in Diabetes Management

Meal planning and portion control are essential components of diabetes management. They play a significant role in regulating blood sugar levels, managing body weight, and preventing complications associated with diabetes. Developing a well-balanced meal plan and practicing portion control empower individuals with diabetes to make healthier food choices and maintain optimal glycemic control. Here's how meal planning and portion control contribute to diabetes management:

Meal Planning:
Meal planning involves creating a structured and balanced eating plan that meets an individual's nutritional needs while managing blood sugar levels. A well-thought-out meal plan helps individuals with diabetes maintain consistent carbohydrate intake, distribute

meals evenly throughout the day, and incorporate a variety of nutrient-rich foods. Here are the key principles of meal planning for diabetes management:

a. **Focus on Nutrient-Dense Foods**: Emphasize nutrient-dense foods such as whole grains, fruits, vegetables, lean proteins, and healthy fats. These foods provide essential vitamins, minerals, and fiber while having a slower impact on blood sugar levels.

b. **Carbohydrate Counting**: Monitor carbohydrate intake by counting grams of carbohydrates in foods. This practice helps individuals match insulin or medication doses with carbohydrate consumption, leading to better blood sugar control.

c. **Consistency in Meal Timing**: Aim to eat meals at regular intervals throughout the day to avoid extreme fluctuations in blood sugar levels. Spacing meals consistently also helps prevent overeating at subsequent meals.

d. **Customize Based on Individual Needs**: Meal plans should be personalized to suit individual preferences, cultural background, activity levels, and type of diabetes. Working with a registered dietitian or diabetes educator can help create a tailored meal plan that aligns with specific health goals.

e. **Include a Variety of Food Groups**: Incorporate foods from all food groups to ensure a balanced intake of nutrients. This includes carbohydrates, proteins, fats, fruits, vegetables, and dairy or dairy alternatives.

Portion Control:
Portion control is the practice of moderating the quantity of food consumed in a single sitting. It helps manage calorie intake, prevents overeating, and contributes to weight management. For individuals with diabetes, portion control is particularly important to prevent large spikes in blood sugar levels.

Here are some strategies for practicing portion control:

a. **Use Smaller Plates**: Using smaller plates and bowls can help control portion sizes and prevent overeating.

b. **Measure Serving Sizes**: Use measuring cups, spoons, and food scales to accurately measure portion sizes, especially for carbohydrate-containing foods.

c. **Be Mindful of Restaurant Portions**: Restaurant meals often contain larger portions than necessary. Consider sharing a meal or asking for a to-go container to save half of the meal for later.

d. **Eat Slowly and Mindfully**: Take time to chew food thoroughly and savor the flavors. Eating slowly can help you recognize feelings of fullness and prevent overeating.

e. **Balance Your Plate**: Aim to fill half of your plate with non-starchy vegetables, one-quarter with lean protein, and one-quarter with whole grains or other carbohydrates.

f. **Plan Snacks Wisely**: Plan snacks in advance and choose nutrient-dense options to avoid mindless snacking on high-calorie, sugary foods.

Both meal planning and portion control complement each other in promoting balanced eating habits and better diabetes management. Consistency in these practices helps stabilize blood sugar levels, maintain a healthy body weight, and reduce the risk of diabetes-related complications. By working with a healthcare team, individuals with diabetes can create effective meal plans and learn portion control techniques tailored to their specific needs and preferences.

Chapter 6: Physical Activity and Diabetes

Benefits of Exercise for Diabetics

Exercise is a powerful tool for managing diabetes and improving overall health. For individuals with diabetes, regular physical activity offers a wide range of benefits that contribute to better glycemic control, weight management, cardiovascular health, and overall well-being. Here are the key benefits of exercise for diabetics:

Improved Blood Sugar Control:
One of the primary benefits of exercise for diabetics is its ability to lower blood sugar levels. During physical activity, muscles use glucose for energy, which helps to reduce blood sugar levels. Regular exercise increases insulin sensitivity, allowing the body to use insulin more effectively, leading to better glycemic control.

Weight Management:
Exercise plays a crucial role in weight management for individuals with diabetes. Engaging in physical activity helps burn calories, promote fat loss, and build lean muscle mass. Achieving and maintaining a healthy weight can improve insulin sensitivity and reduce the risk of obesity-related complications.

Enhanced Insulin Sensitivity:
Regular exercise improves the body's response to insulin, allowing cells to take up glucose more efficiently. This can lead to reduced insulin resistance, a common issue in Type 2 diabetes.

Cardiovascular Health:
Diabetes increases the risk of cardiovascular complications, such as heart disease and stroke. Exercise benefits the cardiovascular system by improving heart function, lowering blood pressure, and increasing HDL (good) cholesterol levels while reducing LDL (bad) cholesterol and triglycerides.

These effects contribute to a healthier heart and reduced risk of cardiovascular disease in individuals with diabetes.

Increased Energy and Endurance:
Regular physical activity can lead to increased energy levels and improved endurance. Individuals with diabetes often report feeling more energetic and capable of handling daily activities with less fatigue.

Stress Reduction:
Exercise is a natural stress reliever. Physical activity stimulates the release of endorphins, which are hormones that improve mood and reduce stress. Managing stress is particularly important for individuals with diabetes, as stress can influence blood sugar levels.

Improved Blood Pressure:
Physical activity helps lower blood pressure, reducing the risk of hypertension and its associated complications.

High blood pressure is common in individuals with diabetes and can increase the risk of heart disease, stroke, and kidney problems.

Better Sleep Quality:
Regular exercise can improve sleep quality and help individuals fall asleep faster. Adequate sleep is crucial for overall health and diabetes management.

Bone Health:
Weight-bearing exercises, such as walking, jogging, or strength training, can promote bone health and reduce the risk of osteoporosis, a condition that weakens bones and increases fracture risk.

Reduced Diabetes Complications:
By managing blood sugar levels, weight, and cardiovascular health, regular exercise can significantly reduce the risk of diabetes-related complications, such as nerve damage (neuropathy), kidney disease (nephropathy), and eye problems (retinopathy).

Before starting an exercise program, individuals with diabetes should consult their healthcare team to determine the most suitable activities and to address any specific considerations or precautions. A mix of aerobic exercises (e.g., walking, swimming, cycling) and strength training can provide comprehensive benefits. The goal is to engage in regular, moderate-intensity exercise for at least 150 minutes per week, with adjustments based on individual fitness levels and health status.

Exercise is a cornerstone of diabetes management that complements other aspects of care, including medication, diet, and blood glucose monitoring. By incorporating regular physical activity into their routines, individuals with diabetes can experience improved blood sugar control, better overall health, and a higher quality of life.

Creating an Exercise Routine Tailored to Individual Needs

Designing a personalized exercise routine is essential for individuals with diabetes as it takes into account their specific health condition, fitness level, preferences, and goals. An exercise plan tailored to individual needs maximizes the benefits of physical activity while minimizing the risk of injury and complications. Here are the steps to create an exercise routine customized for individuals with diabetes:

Consult with Healthcare Professionals: Before starting any exercise program, consult with your healthcare team, including your doctor and diabetes educator. They can provide valuable insights into your overall health, any diabetes-related complications or limitations, and specific exercise recommendations based on your medical history.

Set Realistic Goals:
Determine your exercise goals, considering factors such as improving blood sugar control, managing weight, increasing endurance, or enhancing overall fitness. Set realistic and achievable targets that align with your current fitness level and lifestyle.

Choose Appropriate Activities:
Select activities that you enjoy and are suitable for your fitness level and physical abilities. Aerobic exercises, such as brisk walking, swimming, cycling, dancing, and low-impact aerobics, are generally recommended for individuals with diabetes. These activities help improve cardiovascular health and aid in blood sugar management.

Include Strength Training:
Incorporate strength training exercises, such as weight lifting or bodyweight exercises, into your routine. Strength training helps build lean muscle mass, improves metabolism, and enhances

overall functional fitness. It can also have a positive impact on blood sugar control and insulin sensitivity.

Consider Flexibility and Balance Exercises:
Include flexibility and balance exercises in your routine to improve joint mobility, reduce the risk of falls, and enhance overall body coordination. Activities like yoga, tai chi, or stretching exercises can be beneficial.

Warm-Up and Cool Down:
Always begin your exercise routine with a proper warm-up to increase blood flow to muscles and prepare your body for physical activity. Similarly, end each session with a cool-down and stretching to reduce muscle soreness and promote flexibility.

Monitor Blood Sugar Levels:
Regularly check your blood sugar levels before, during, and after exercise, especially if you take insulin or certain

diabetes medications. Monitoring helps
you understand how exercise affects your
blood sugar levels and allows you to
adjust your routine accordingly.

Consider Time and Frequency:
Gradually build up the duration and
intensity of your workouts. Aim for at
least 150 minutes of moderate-intensity
aerobic exercise per week, spread across
several days. You can break down the
sessions into shorter bouts to make it more
manageable.

Stay Hydrated:
Stay well-hydrated during exercise,
especially if you engage in activities that
cause sweating. Drink water before,
during, and after your workouts.

Listen to Your Body:
Be mindful of how your body responds to
exercise. If you experience discomfort,
pain, or dizziness, stop the activity and
consult your healthcare team.

Adjust for Special Circumstances:
Consider how factors such as travel, illness, or changes in your routine may impact your exercise plan. Be flexible and adapt your routine as needed to maintain consistency.

Track Progress:
Keep a log of your exercise sessions, including the type of activity, duration, and any observations about your blood sugar responses or overall well-being. Tracking progress can help you stay motivated and identify patterns or improvements over time.

Remember that individual needs and preferences may evolve over time, so periodically reassess your exercise routine and make adjustments as necessary. Creating an exercise routine tailored to your individual needs empowers you to experience the full benefits of physical activity while effectively managing diabetes and improving your overall health and well-being.

Safe Exercises for Different Age Groups and

Fitness Levels

Tailoring exercise routines to individual age groups and fitness levels is crucial to ensure safety, prevent injuries, and promote overall well-being. Here are some safe exercise options for different age groups and fitness levels:

Children and Adolescents (Age 6 to 17): Children and adolescents should engage in physical activities that support their growth and development while being enjoyable and age-appropriate. Focus on activities that encourage movement, coordination, and social interaction:

Active Play: Encourage unstructured play, such as running, jumping, climbing, and playing sports, to develop motor skills and build strength and endurance.

Team Sports: Participate in team sports like soccer, basketball, or volleyball, which promote teamwork and physical fitness.

Swimming: Swimming is an excellent full-body exercise that is low-impact and suitable for all ages.

Dance: Dance classes or activities like Zumba can be enjoyable ways for children and teens to stay active.

Young Adults (Age 18 to 35): Young adults have the flexibility to explore various exercise options to improve their fitness level and overall health:

Cardiovascular Exercises: Engage in activities like running, cycling, or aerobic classes to improve cardiovascular endurance.

Strength Training: Incorporate resistance training using free weights, machines, or bodyweight exercises to build lean muscle mass and improve metabolism.

High-Intensity Interval Training (HIIT): HIIT workouts involve short bursts of intense exercise followed by brief rest periods and can be effective for time-efficient workouts.

Yoga and Pilates: These activities can improve flexibility, balance, and core strength.

Adults (Age 36 to 64):
For adults, maintaining a balanced exercise routine is important to support overall health and manage stress:

Moderate Cardiovascular Exercise: Activities like brisk walking, swimming, or cycling provide cardiovascular benefits without excessive impact.

Strength Training: Continue with resistance training to preserve muscle mass and bone density.

Flexibility and Balance Exercises: Include stretching, yoga, or tai chi to maintain flexibility and reduce the risk of falls.

Low-Impact Exercises: Engage in low-impact options like elliptical training or water aerobics to protect joints.

Older Adults (Age 65 and above): Older adults should focus on exercises that promote functional fitness, maintain independence, and reduce the risk of falls:

Walking: Regular walking is a safe and effective way to improve cardiovascular health and maintain mobility.

Chair Exercises: Exercises performed while seated can help maintain muscle strength and flexibility.

Balance and Stability Exercises: Tai chi, yoga, and specific balance exercises can improve stability and reduce the risk of falls.

Water Exercises: Water aerobics or swimming in a heated pool can be gentle on joints while providing resistance for muscle strengthening.

Safety Tips for All Age Groups: *Regardless of age, it is essential to consider safety when engaging in physical activity*:

Warm-Up and Cool-Down: Always warm up before exercise and cool down afterward to prevent injuries.

Listen to Your Body: Pay attention to any pain or discomfort during exercise and stop if something doesn't feel right.

Stay Hydrated: Drink plenty of water before, during, and after exercise to avoid dehydration.

Start Slowly: If you are new to exercise or returning after a break, start with low-intensity activities and gradually increase the intensity and duration.

Include Rest Days: Allow your body time to recover by incorporating rest days into your exercise routine.

Consult a Healthcare Professional: Before starting a new exercise program, consult with your doctor or healthcare provider, especially if you have any pre-existing medical conditions or concerns.

By choosing safe and age-appropriate exercises, individuals can enjoy the numerous benefits of physical activity while reducing the risk of injuries and maintaining their overall health and well-being at every stage of life.

Overview of Diabetes Medications and Their

Mechanisms

Diabetes medications are used to help manage blood sugar levels in individuals with diabetes. The choice of medication depends on the type of diabetes, individual health needs, and response to other diabetes management strategies such as diet and exercise. Here's an overview of the main classes of diabetes medications and their mechanisms of action:

Insulin:
Insulin is a hormone produced by the pancreas that regulates blood sugar levels by facilitating the uptake of glucose into cells for energy. In Type 1 diabetes and some cases of Type 2 diabetes, the body does not produce enough insulin or cannot effectively use it.

Insulin therapy is the primary treatment for Type 1 diabetes and may be prescribed for some individuals with Type 2 diabetes. It is usually administered through injections or insulin pumps.

Metformin:
Metformin is the first-line medication for most individuals with Type 2 diabetes. It belongs to the biguanide class of medications and works by reducing glucose production in the liver and improving insulin sensitivity in the muscles and tissues. Metformin also slows down the absorption of glucose from the intestines.

Sulfonylureas:
Sulfonylureas are oral medications that stimulate the pancreas to produce more insulin. They are primarily used in Type 2 diabetes when lifestyle changes and metformin are insufficient to control blood sugar levels. Examples of sulfonylureas include glipizide, glyburide, and glimepiride.

Meglitinides:
Meglitinides are oral medications that also stimulate insulin secretion from the pancreas, but they have a shorter duration of action compared to sulfonylureas. They are typically taken before meals to help control post-meal blood sugar spikes. Examples include repaglinide and nateglinide.

Dipeptidyl Peptidase-4 (DPP-4) Inhibitors:
DPP-4 inhibitors are oral medications that work by blocking the enzyme DPP-4, which degrades incretin hormones. These hormones stimulate insulin release and inhibit glucagon secretion, leading to lower blood sugar levels. DPP-4 inhibitors include sitagliptin, saxagliptin, linagliptin, and alogliptin.

Sodium-Glucose Co-Transporter 2 (SGLT-2) Inhibitors:
SGLT-2 inhibitors are a newer class of medications that reduce blood sugar levels by blocking the reabsorption of glucose in

the kidneys, leading to increased urinary excretion of glucose. This class includes drugs like canagliflozin, dapagliflozin, and empagliflozin.

Glucagon-Like Peptide-1 (GLP-1) Receptor Agonists:
GLP-1 receptor agonists are injectable medications that mimic the action of GLP-1, an incretin hormone that stimulates insulin secretion and suppresses glucagon release. These medications also slow down gastric emptying, leading to a feeling of fullness and reduced appetite. GLP-1 receptor agonists include exenatide, liraglutide, dulaglutide, and semaglutide.

Thiazolidinediones (TZDs):
TZDs are oral medications that improve insulin sensitivity in muscle and adipose tissue, thereby reducing insulin resistance. They are typically used in Type 2 diabetes when other medications are not effective or tolerated. Examples of TZDs include pioglitazone and rosiglitazone.

Alpha-Glucosidase Inhibitors:
Alpha-glucosidase inhibitors work by delaying the breakdown and absorption of carbohydrates in the intestines, leading to a slower rise in blood sugar after meals. Acarbose and miglitol are examples of alpha-glucosidase inhibitors.

Bile Acid Sequestrants:
Bile acid sequestrants are used to treat both Type 2 diabetes and certain lipid disorders. They work by binding to bile acids in the intestines, which helps lower blood sugar levels by an unknown mechanism.

It's important to note that the choice of diabetes medication and its mechanism of action may vary depending on individual health factors, preferences, and the specific type of diabetes being treated. Medication management should always be done under the supervision and guidance of healthcare professionals, and regular monitoring of blood sugar levels is essential to ensure optimal diabetes management. Additionally, lifestyle changes, including diet, exercise, and weight management, are crucial components of diabetes care and may be used alone or in combination with medications to achieve optimal blood sugar control.

Insulin Therapy and Delivery Methods

Insulin therapy is a crucial aspect of diabetes management, primarily used for individuals with Type 1 diabetes and some cases of Type 2 diabetes where oral medications are insufficient to control blood sugar levels. Insulin therapy aims to mimic the body's natural production of insulin to regulate blood glucose effectively. There are several delivery methods for administering insulin, each offering unique advantages and considerations. Here's an overview of insulin therapy and its various delivery methods:

Insulin Injection Pens:
Insulin pens are one of the most common and convenient methods of insulin delivery. They resemble writing pens and come pre-filled with insulin cartridges or as disposable, prefilled pens. Some insulin pens are reusable and allow the attachment of replaceable insulin cartridges.

Advantages: Easy to use, discreet, and portable. Dosing is accurate, making them suitable for precise insulin delivery.

Considerations: Different pens may require specific types of insulin cartridges, and they can be relatively more expensive than vials of insulin.

Insulin Syringes:
Insulin syringes are traditional devices used to draw insulin from vials and inject it subcutaneously (under the skin). They consist of a needle and a barrel with volume markings to measure the insulin dose.
Advantages: Cost-effective, widely available, and suitable for those who prefer a more hands-on approach to insulin administration.

Considerations: May require more manual dexterity, and dosing accuracy may vary based on the user's skill.

Insulin Pumps:
Insulin pumps are small devices that deliver insulin continuously through a tiny, flexible tube (catheter) inserted under the skin. The pump is worn on the body and is programmed to provide a basal (background) insulin rate throughout the day, with additional bolus doses before meals.

Advantages: Offers precise insulin delivery, allows for flexibility in basal rates, and facilitates precise bolus dosing for mealtime insulin needs. Reduces the number of injections required.

Considerations: Requires regular maintenance and monitoring of blood glucose levels to adjust pump settings. It involves wearing a device on the body continuously.

Insulin Jet Injectors:
Insulin jet injectors use a high-pressure stream of insulin to penetrate the skin, delivering insulin without a needle.

The insulin is delivered in a fine spray through the skin.

Advantages: Needle-free delivery, which can be beneficial for individuals with needle phobia or those who have difficulty using traditional injection methods.

Considerations: May be less accurate in insulin dosing compared to other delivery methods. Currently, jet injectors are less commonly used.

Inhaled Insulin:
Inhaled insulin involves delivering insulin into the lungs using a specialized inhaler. The insulin is absorbed through the lung tissues into the bloodstream.

Advantages: Needle-free, quick absorption, and convenient for certain individuals.

Considerations: Inhaled insulin is currently limited to specific formulations and may not be suitable for everyone, particularly those with certain respiratory conditions.

The choice of insulin delivery method depends on factors such as individual preference, lifestyle, treatment goals, and healthcare provider recommendations. Healthcare professionals work with individuals to determine the most suitable insulin regimen and delivery method based on their specific needs and medical history. Regular monitoring of blood sugar levels and consistent adherence to the insulin therapy plan are crucial for optimal diabetes management and overall well-being.

Insulin is a life-saving medication used to manage diabetes, and it is essential to handle and store it correctly to ensure its effectiveness and safety. Proper administration and storage of insulin play a vital role in maintaining its potency and reducing the risk of adverse effects. Here are guidelines for the proper administration and storage of insulin:

Insulin Administration:
a. **Injection Site**: Insulin is typically injected subcutaneously, which means it is injected into the fatty tissue just under the skin. Common injection sites include the abdomen, thighs, buttocks, and upper arms. Rotate injection sites within the same general area to prevent lipohypertrophy (thickened fatty tissue) and ensure consistent absorption.

b. **Needle Size**: Use the appropriate needle size for insulin injections. Needle lengths vary, but shorter, finer needles are often more comfortable and reduce the risk of injecting into muscle.

c. **Injection Technique**: Inject insulin at a 90-degree angle if using a shorter needle or at a 45-degree angle if using a longer needle or if you have reduced fatty tissue. Follow proper injection techniques to ensure accurate dosing and minimize discomfort.

d. **Insulin Pens and Syringes**: If using insulin pens or syringes, follow the manufacturer's instructions for their proper use and storage.

e. **Insulin Pumps**: If using an insulin pump, carefully follow the manufacturer's instructions for insertion, programming, and management of the pump.

Insulin Storage:
a. **Temperature**: Store insulin at the recommended temperature range, typically between 36°F to 46°F (2°C to 8°C).

Never freeze insulin, as it can lose its effectiveness when thawed. Insulin that has been frozen should be discarded.

b. **Unopened Insulin**: Unopened insulin vials, cartridges, or pens should be stored in the refrigerator until the expiration date on the package. Always check the expiration date before using any insulin product.

c. **Room Temperature**: Insulin that is currently being used can be kept at room temperature (between 59°F to 86°F or 15°C to 30°C) for up to 28 days. However, it is essential to protect insulin from direct sunlight and extreme heat. Avoid leaving insulin in a hot car or direct sunlight, as it can degrade the insulin.

d. **Insulin in Use**: If keeping insulin at room temperature, write the date it was removed from the refrigerator on the insulin vial or pen. Discard any insulin that has been kept at room temperature for more than 28 days.

e. **Avoid Extreme Temperatures**: Do not expose insulin to extreme temperatures, such as leaving it in a hot or freezing-cold environment, as it can lead to degradation and loss of effectiveness.

Check for Changes:
Before each use, inspect the insulin for any changes in appearance, such as clumping, discoloration, or particles. If you notice any abnormalities, do not use the insulin, and contact your healthcare provider or pharmacist for a replacement.

Traveling with Insulin:
When traveling, carry insulin in a cooler bag with ice packs to maintain the proper temperature. Avoid storing insulin directly on ice, as it can freeze and become ineffective.

Always consult with your healthcare provider or diabetes educator for specific instructions on insulin administration and storage.

Following these guidelines will help ensure the insulin's potency, effectiveness, and safety, contributing to better diabetes management and overall health.

Common complications of uncontrolled diabetes

Uncontrolled diabetes, whether it is Type 1 or Type 2, can lead to various complications that affect multiple organ systems in the body. Consistently high blood sugar levels can damage blood vessels and nerves, contributing to the development of long-term complications. Proper diabetes management is essential to reduce the risk of these complications. Here are some common complications of uncontrolled diabetes:

Cardiovascular Complications:
Atherosclerosis: Uncontrolled diabetes can lead to the development of atherosclerosis, a condition where the blood vessels become narrowed and hardened due to the accumulation of plaque.

Atherosclerosis increases the risk of heart attacks, strokes, and peripheral artery disease (PAD).

Hypertension (High Blood Pressure): High blood sugar levels can damage the blood vessels, leading to increased blood pressure, which further raises the risk of cardiovascular events.

Diabetic Retinopathy: Diabetic retinopathy is a complication that affects the eyes and is a leading cause of blindness in adults. Prolonged high blood sugar levels damage the blood vessels in the retina, leading to vision problems and potentially irreversible vision loss.

Diabetic Neuropathy: Diabetic neuropathy is nerve damage caused by chronic high blood sugar levels. It most commonly affects the feet and legs, leading to symptoms such as tingling, numbness, burning sensations, and loss of sensation. Severe cases of neuropathy can cause pain and impair mobility.

Diabetic Nephropathy:
Uncontrolled diabetes can damage the
small blood vessels in the kidneys, leading
to diabetic nephropathy. It is a progressive
kidney disease that may result in reduced
kidney function and, in severe cases, end-
stage renal disease (ESRD) requiring
dialysis or kidney transplant.

Diabetic Foot Ulcers:
Nerve damage and poor blood circulation
in the feet can result in foot complications,
such as diabetic foot ulcers. These ulcers
are slow-healing wounds that can lead to
infections and, in severe cases, may
require amputation.

Peripheral Neuropathy:
Besides affecting the feet and legs,
diabetic neuropathy can also involve other
peripheral nerves in the body. This can
lead to digestive issues, sexual
dysfunction, and problems with the
autonomic nervous system, which controls
involuntary bodily functions like blood
pressure and heart rate.

Skin Complications:
Uncontrolled diabetes can lead to various skin conditions, including bacterial and fungal infections, as well as slow-healing wounds.

Dental Complications:
Diabetes increases the risk of gum disease (periodontitis) and other dental problems due to the impaired ability to fight off bacterial infections.

Increased Susceptibility to Infections:
High blood sugar levels can weaken the immune system, making individuals with diabetes more susceptible to infections, especially those affecting the urinary tract, skin, and respiratory system.

Mental Health Issues:
Managing diabetes can be challenging, and the chronic nature of the condition can lead to stress, anxiety, and depression in some individuals.

Preventing or minimizing these complications involves maintaining good blood sugar control, adopting a healthy lifestyle, regularly monitoring blood sugar levels, taking medications as prescribed, and working closely with a healthcare team to manage diabetes effectively. Early detection and prompt management of any complications that arise are essential to prevent further progression and maintain the best possible quality of life for individuals living with diabetes.

Preventing and managing complications associated with diabetes is crucial to maintaining good health and well-being for individuals living with the condition. Proper diabetes management involves a combination of lifestyle changes, regular medical care, and adherence to treatment plans. Here are some effective strategies to prevent and manage complications of diabetes:

Blood Sugar Control:
Maintaining stable blood sugar levels is essential to prevent or delay diabetes-related complications. Consistently high blood sugar levels can lead to damage to blood vessels and nerves throughout the body.
Follow these steps to achieve better blood sugar control:

Monitor Blood Sugar: Regularly check blood sugar levels as recommended by your healthcare team, and adjust insulin or medication doses accordingly.

Follow a Meal Plan: Work with a registered dietitian or diabetes educator to create a personalized meal plan that helps manage blood sugar levels and supports overall health.

Engage in Physical Activity: Incorporate regular exercise into your routine, as it can improve insulin sensitivity and help regulate blood sugar levels.

Take Medications as Prescribed: Follow your healthcare provider's instructions for taking diabetes medications, including insulin, oral medications, or other prescribed treatments.

Regular Medical Check-ups: Regular medical check-ups and screenings are essential to monitor and manage diabetes-related complications.

Your healthcare team can detect early signs of complications and take appropriate actions to prevent their progression. Schedule regular visits with your doctor, eye doctor, dentist, and other specialists as recommended.

Blood Pressure and Cholesterol Management:
High blood pressure and cholesterol are risk factors for cardiovascular complications in individuals with diabetes. Follow a heart-healthy lifestyle, take prescribed medications as directed, and work with your healthcare provider to control blood pressure and cholesterol levels.

Stop Smoking:
If you smoke, quitting is one of the most significant steps you can take to prevent complications of diabetes. Smoking can further damage blood vessels and exacerbate the risks of cardiovascular issues.

Foot Care:
Take care of your feet to prevent complications such as diabetic foot ulcers and infections. Inspect your feet regularly for any wounds or abnormalities, keep your feet clean and dry, and wear comfortable, well-fitting shoes and socks.

Eye Health:
Schedule regular eye exams with an eye care professional to monitor and manage diabetic retinopathy and other eye-related complications.

Kidney Health:
Manage blood pressure and blood sugar levels to protect kidney function. Regularly monitor kidney function through urine tests and blood tests as recommended by your healthcare provider.

Dental Care:
Practice good oral hygiene and visit the dentist regularly for check-ups and cleanings to prevent dental complications associated with diabetes.

Stress Management:
Chronic stress can affect blood sugar levels and overall health. Find stress-relief techniques that work for you, such as exercise, meditation, yoga, or spending time with loved ones.

Diabetes Education and Support:
Participate in diabetes education programs to improve your understanding of diabetes management and how to prevent complications. Support from diabetes educators, support groups, and online communities can provide valuable insights and motivation.

Stay Informed:
Stay up-to-date with the latest advancements in diabetes management and be proactive in discussing new treatment options with your healthcare team.

Remember that diabetes is a chronic condition that requires ongoing management.

With proper self-care, adherence to medical advice, and a strong support system, individuals with diabetes can reduce the risk of complications and lead a healthy and fulfilling life. Always consult with your healthcare provider to develop a comprehensive plan tailored to your specific health needs and goals.

The Importance of Regular Check-ups and Screenings

Regular check-ups and screenings are crucial for maintaining good health and detecting potential health issues early, including those related to diabetes. For individuals living with diabetes, these routine medical visits play an even more critical role in preventing complications and optimizing disease management. Here are several reasons highlighting the importance of regular check-ups and screenings for individuals with diabetes:

Early Detection of Complications: Regular check-ups allow healthcare professionals to monitor your overall health and assess diabetes-related complications. Early detection of complications such as diabetic retinopathy, neuropathy, nephropathy, cardiovascular issues, and foot problems enables timely intervention and management, which can help prevent or delay the progression of these conditions.

Blood Sugar Control and Medication Adjustments:
During check-ups, your healthcare provider will review your blood sugar levels and assess the effectiveness of your diabetes management plan. They may make necessary adjustments to your medication regimen, insulin doses, or other treatment strategies based on your blood sugar trends and health status.

Assessment of Risk Factors:
Health check-ups provide an opportunity to assess your risk factors for various conditions, including cardiovascular disease. Identifying risk factors such as high blood pressure, high cholesterol, and obesity allows your healthcare team to implement preventive measures and address these factors before they lead to more serious complications.

Evaluation of Lifestyle Habits:
Regular check-ups offer an opportunity to discuss your lifestyle habits with your healthcare provider. They can provide guidance on maintaining a healthy diet, incorporating regular exercise, quitting smoking, and managing stress—all of which play crucial roles in diabetes management and overall health.

Monitoring Blood Pressure and Cholesterol:
Individuals with diabetes are at an increased risk of developing hypertension (high blood pressure) and dyslipidemia (abnormal cholesterol levels). Regular check-ups help monitor and manage these conditions, reducing the risk of cardiovascular complications associated with diabetes.

Eye Examinations:
Routine eye exams are essential for individuals with diabetes to monitor eye health and detect diabetic retinopathy or other eye-related complications early.

Early detection and treatment can help preserve vision and prevent severe eye problems.

Kidney Function Assessment:
Check-ups include testing kidney function through urine tests and blood tests. These assessments help identify any signs of kidney damage (diabetic nephropathy) and enable timely intervention to protect kidney health.

Foot Care:
Healthcare providers can conduct foot examinations during check-ups to identify any foot problems or early signs of diabetic foot ulcers. Regular foot care and preventive measures can help prevent serious foot complications and reduce the risk of amputations.

Emotional Support and Education:
Check-ups provide opportunities for diabetes education, support, and counseling. Healthcare professionals can address any concerns or emotional

challenges related to diabetes, offering guidance and support to cope with the demands of living with a chronic condition.

Empowerment and Partnership: Regular check-ups allow you to actively engage in your diabetes management. By discussing your progress and goals with your healthcare team, you become an informed and empowered partner in your own healthcare journey.

Regular check-ups and screenings are essential components of diabetes care. They provide a comprehensive assessment of your health, facilitate early detection of complications, and support ongoing diabetes management. By attending these appointments and working closely with your healthcare team, you can take proactive steps to protect your health, optimize diabetes management, and enhance your overall well-being.

Chapter 9: Living Well with Diabetes

Coping with the Emotional Aspects of Diabetes

Living with diabetes can be challenging, and it's essential to recognize and address the emotional aspects that come with managing a chronic condition. The emotional impact of diabetes can vary from person to person, and individuals may experience a range of feelings such as stress, anxiety, fear, frustration, and even depression. Coping with the emotional aspects of diabetes is crucial for overall well-being and effective diabetes management. Here are some strategies to help individuals navigate and cope with the emotional aspects of diabetes:

Education and Awareness:
One of the first steps in coping with diabetes emotionally is to gain a deeper

understanding of the condition. Learn about diabetes, its management, potential complications, and treatment options. Knowledge empowers individuals to take control of their health and make informed decisions about their diabetes care.

Open Communication:
Share your feelings and concerns with your healthcare team, family, and friends. Communicating openly about your emotions can help you feel supported and understood. Your healthcare team can also provide guidance on managing the emotional impact of diabetes.

Support System:
Build a strong support system of family members, friends, and peers who understand and empathize with your diabetes journey. Joining diabetes support groups or online communities can provide valuable emotional support and opportunities to share experiences.

Set Realistic Goals:
Set achievable goals for diabetes management and celebrate small victories. Acknowledge that managing diabetes is a continuous process, and progress may not always be linear. Setting realistic goals can help reduce feelings of overwhelm and anxiety.

Stress Management:
Stress can affect blood sugar levels and overall health. Engage in stress-relief techniques such as exercise, meditation, deep breathing, yoga, or spending time in nature. Finding activities that promote relaxation and mindfulness can help manage stress effectively.

Diabetes Education and Self-Care:
Take advantage of diabetes education programs and resources to improve your self-care skills. Learning how to manage diabetes effectively can increase confidence and reduce feelings of uncertainty.

Focus on Positives:
Rather than dwelling on the challenges of diabetes, focus on the positive aspects of your life. Engage in activities that bring joy, gratitude, and fulfillment.

Seek Professional Help:
If feelings of sadness, anxiety, or depression persist, consider seeking support from a mental health professional. Therapy or counseling can provide valuable tools to cope with emotional challenges and develop resilience.

Address Fear and Anxiety:
Many individuals with diabetes may fear complications or worry about hypoglycemic episodes. Talk to your healthcare team about managing these concerns and develop an action plan to address potential emergencies.

Acceptance and Self-Compassion:
Accept that living with diabetes involves ups and downs. Be kind to yourself and practice self-compassion.

Understand that it's okay to have difficult days and that you are doing your best to manage your health.

Remember that coping with the emotional aspects of diabetes is an ongoing process, and it's okay to seek help and support when needed. By addressing the emotional impact of diabetes and incorporating strategies to promote well-being, individuals can lead fulfilling lives while effectively managing their diabetes.

Lifestyle Adjustments for Better Diabetes Management

Managing diabetes effectively requires a comprehensive approach that includes lifestyle adjustments to maintain stable blood sugar levels, promote overall health, and prevent complications. By making positive changes in daily habits, individuals with diabetes can improve their quality of life and better manage the condition. Here are key lifestyle adjustments for better diabetes management:

Balanced and Healthy Diet:
Adopting a balanced and healthy diet is fundamental to diabetes management. Focus on nutrient-dense foods that support stable blood sugar levels, weight management, and overall health. Key dietary considerations include:

Carbohydrate Management: Monitor carbohydrate intake and choose complex carbohydrates with a low glycemic index, which have a slower impact on blood sugar levels. Spread carbohydrate intake throughout the day to avoid large spikes in blood sugar.

Portion Control: Be mindful of portion sizes to avoid overeating and help regulate blood sugar levels.

Include Protein and Healthy Fats: Protein and healthy fats can help stabilize blood sugar levels and keep you feeling full longer. Include sources such as lean meats, fish, nuts, seeds, avocados, and olive oil in your diet.

Limit Processed Foods and Sugary Beverages: Minimize consumption of sugary foods, processed snacks, and sugary beverages, as they can cause rapid spikes in blood sugar.

Regular Physical Activity:
Regular exercise plays a vital role in diabetes management. Physical activity helps improve insulin sensitivity, maintain a healthy weight, and reduce the risk of cardiovascular complications. Aim for at least 150 minutes of moderate-intensity aerobic exercise, such as brisk walking, swimming, or cycling, per week. Additionally, include strength training exercises at least two days a week to build and maintain muscle mass.

Weight Management:
For those who are overweight or obese, achieving and maintaining a healthy weight is crucial for diabetes management. Losing excess weight can improve insulin sensitivity and blood sugar control. Work with a healthcare provider or a registered dietitian to develop a personalized weight management plan.

Regular Blood Sugar Monitoring:
Frequent monitoring of blood sugar levels provides valuable information for

managing diabetes effectively. Your healthcare provider can help you establish a monitoring schedule and interpret the results to make necessary adjustments to your treatment plan.

Medication Adherence:
Follow your healthcare provider's instructions regarding medication use, including insulin injections or oral medications. Adhering to your prescribed medication regimen is essential for blood sugar control and preventing complications.

Stress Reduction:
Chronic stress can impact blood sugar levels and overall well-being. Engage in stress-reduction techniques such as mindfulness, meditation, yoga, deep breathing, or spending time in nature.

Regular Sleep Patterns:
Adequate and regular sleep is essential for managing diabetes. Aim for 7-9 hours of

quality sleep each night to support overall health and blood sugar control

Regular Medical Check-ups:
Regular visits to your healthcare provider are essential for monitoring your diabetes, identifying potential complications, and making necessary adjustments to your treatment plan.

Avoid Smoking and Limit Alcohol:
Smoking can worsen diabetes complications, while alcohol consumption can affect blood sugar levels. Quitting smoking and limiting alcohol intake are beneficial lifestyle adjustments for better diabetes management.

Diabetes Education and Support:
Participate in diabetes education programs and seek support from healthcare providers, diabetes educators, and support groups. Learning more about diabetes management and connecting with others who share similar experiences can provide

valuable knowledge and emotional support.

By incorporating these lifestyle adjustments into daily routines, individuals with diabetes can take an active role in their health, improve diabetes management, and reduce the risk of complications. It's essential to work closely with a healthcare team to develop a personalized diabetes care plan that meets individual needs and goals.

Tips for managing diabetes during special circumstances

Managing diabetes during special circumstances, such as travel or illness, requires careful planning and flexibility to ensure optimal blood sugar control and overall well-being. Changes in routine, time zones, and eating patterns can affect blood sugar levels, and illness can have additional implications on diabetes management. Here are some practical tips for managing diabetes during special circumstances:

Travel:
Plan Ahead: Before traveling, consult with your healthcare provider to ensure your diabetes is well-managed. Get necessary prescriptions and a letter explaining your medical condition and the supplies you carry (insulin, syringes, etc.) for airport security.

Carry Supplies: Pack extra diabetes supplies, including insulin, test strips, glucose meters, and medications. Keep them in your carry-on bag to avoid any issues if your checked luggage is delayed or lost.

Time Zone Adjustments: If traveling across time zones, work with your healthcare provider to adjust your insulin dosing schedule accordingly. You may need to gradually shift your meal and insulin timings.

Monitor Blood Sugar Frequently: Check your blood sugar levels more frequently than usual, especially during long flights or extended periods of travel. Changes in activity levels and meal times can impact blood sugar.

Stay Hydrated: Drink plenty of water during travel, and avoid sugary or alcoholic beverages that can cause fluctuations in blood sugar levels.

Be Prepared for Emergencies: Carry a glucagon kit (if applicable) and have a plan in case of hypoglycemia or other diabetes-related emergencies.

Illness:

Stay Hydrated: Drink plenty of fluids, especially if you have high blood sugar levels or experience fever, vomiting, or diarrhea. Dehydration can worsen blood sugar control.

Monitor Blood Sugar and Ketones: Test your blood sugar levels more frequently when you're sick. If you have Type 1 diabetes, check for ketones in your urine or blood, especially if your blood sugar levels are consistently high.

Continue Insulin and Medications: Even when you're ill and not eating much, it's crucial to continue taking your insulin or diabetes medications as prescribed.

Eat Small, Frequent Meals: If you have a reduced appetite, try to eat small, nutrient-dense meals throughout the day to maintain blood sugar levels.

Have a Sick-Day Plan: Work with your healthcare provider to develop a sick-day plan that includes specific guidelines for managing your diabetes during illness, including medication adjustments if needed.

Seek Medical Attention: Contact your healthcare provider if you experience severe or prolonged illness or if you have difficulty managing your blood sugar levels.

Special Events or Holidays:

Plan Meals Ahead: If attending special events or holidays, plan your meals in advance and consider the carbohydrate content of the dishes you'll be eating.

Be Mindful of Alcohol: If consuming alcohol, do so in moderation and consider its impact on blood sugar levels.

Stay Active: Engage in physical activity or take a walk after meals to help manage blood sugar levels.

Stay Connected: Inform friends and family about your diabetes, so they can support your needs during special events or gatherings.

Remember, diabetes management is a continuous process, and special circumstances may require additional attention and adjustments. Flexibility and preparation are essential in maintaining stable blood sugar levels and overall health during travel, illness, or special events. Always communicate with your healthcare provider for personalized advice and guidance in managing diabetes during these unique situations.

Current trends in diabetes research

Continuous Glucose Monitoring (CGM) Technology:

Continuous Glucose Monitoring (CGM) systems were gaining popularity for diabetes management. CGMs offer real-time monitoring of glucose levels, providing users with more comprehensive data to make informed decisions about insulin dosing, diet, and physical activity. Researchers were working on enhancing CGM accuracy and exploring new ways to integrate CGM data with insulin pumps and artificial pancreas systems.

Closed-Loop Systems (Artificial Pancreas):

Closed-loop systems, also known as artificial pancreas systems, combine CGM technology with insulin pumps to automate insulin delivery based on real-time glucose data. These systems aim to provide better glucose control and reduce the burden of diabetes management. Research was ongoing to improve the safety and efficacy of closed-loop systems, especially for use in different age groups and during specific circumstances, such as exercise or illness.

Insulin Delivery Systems:
Researchers were investigating alternative insulin delivery methods, such as inhaled insulin and oral insulin, to offer more options for people who require insulin therapy. Inhaled insulin had already been approved for use, and oral insulin was being explored as a potential non-injectable option.

Personalized Medicine and Precision Therapies:
Advancements in genetics and personalized medicine were starting to influence diabetes research.

Scientists were studying genetic factors that contribute to the development of diabetes and tailoring treatment plans based on an individual's genetic profile. Precision therapies were being explored to target specific aspects of diabetes based on a person's unique needs and characteristics.

Immunotherapies for Type 1 Diabetes: Research was ongoing to develop immunotherapies that could prevent or delay the autoimmune destruction of insulin-producing beta cells in Type 1 diabetes. These therapies aim to preserve or restore insulin production and potentially halt the progression of the disease.

Gut Microbiome and Diabetes: Scientists were investigating the role of the gut microbiome in diabetes. Emerging research suggested that the composition of gut bacteria might influence insulin sensitivity and glucose regulation.

Understanding this link could lead to new approaches in diabetes prevention and management.

Lifestyle Interventions:
Studies were examining the impact of lifestyle interventions, such as diet and exercise, in preventing or managing diabetes. Researchers were investigating specific dietary patterns (e.g., Mediterranean diet, low-carbohydrate diet) and the benefits of different exercise regimens on blood sugar control.

Diabetes Technology and Mobile Apps:
The development of diabetes-related mobile apps and digital health tools was gaining momentum. These apps offered features like meal tracking, glucose monitoring, and medication reminders, aiming to empower individuals with diabetes to manage their condition more effectively.

It's important to note that diabetes research is an ever-evolving field, and new discoveries and breakthroughs are continually emerging. Ongoing research and advancements in diabetes management hold the potential to improve the lives of millions of individuals living with diabetes worldwide. For the latest updates and current trends in diabetes research, it is best to consult recent publications and trusted medical sources.

Closed-Loop Systems and Artificial Pancreas:

Closed-loop systems, also known as artificial pancreas systems, were gaining momentum as a cutting-edge technology for diabetes management. These systems combine continuous glucose monitoring (CGM) with insulin pumps to automate insulin delivery based on real-time glucose data. Closed-loop systems aim to provide more precise and stable blood sugar control, reducing the need for manual adjustments and enhancing overall diabetes management.

Insulin Pump Technology:

Advancements in insulin pump technology were underway, making these devices smaller, more discreet, and user-friendly. New features were being developed to improve insulin delivery accuracy, provide more data insights, and integrate with other diabetes technologies like CGM systems.

Glucose-Sensing Contact Lenses: Researchers were exploring the use of contact lenses with built-in glucose sensors to continuously monitor blood sugar levels through tears. This innovative technology could offer a non-invasive and convenient method for people with diabetes to monitor their glucose levels in real-time.

Oral Insulin: Oral insulin was a promising area of research that sought to provide an alternative to injectable insulin for individuals with diabetes. Scientists were working to develop oral insulin formulations that could survive the digestive process and be effectively absorbed into the bloodstream to manage blood sugar levels.

Islet Cell Transplantation:
Islet cell transplantation continued to show promise as a potential treatment for Type 1 diabetes. Researchers were investigating ways to improve the success and long-term viability of islet cell transplants to restore insulin production in individuals with Type 1 diabetes.

Gene Therapy and Immunotherapy:
Gene therapy and immunotherapy approaches were being explored to address the underlying causes of diabetes. These innovative treatments aimed to target the immune system's response in Type 1 diabetes or modify genes related to insulin sensitivity in Type 2 diabetes.

Smart Insulin:
Smart insulin technology involved developing insulin formulations that respond to blood sugar levels, releasing insulin only when needed. These smart insulin products aimed to mimic the function of the pancreas more closely,

leading to improved glucose control and reduced risk of hypoglycemia.

Advanced Diabetes Data Analytics: Advancements in data analytics and artificial intelligence were being utilized to analyze large volumes of diabetes-related data, such as glucose levels, dietary habits, and physical activity. These analytics aimed to provide personalized insights and recommendations for diabetes management, helping individuals make informed decisions about their health.

It's important to note that while these treatments and technologies showed promise in research and clinical trials, further studies, regulatory approvals, and real-world applications are necessary to establish their safety, efficacy, and accessibility. The landscape of diabetes research is continuously evolving, and ongoing efforts are directed toward improving diabetes care and finding innovative solutions to better manage this chronic condition.

For the latest updates on promising treatments and technologies, it is best to consult recent scientific literature and reputable medical sources.

Advocating for diabetes awareness and support

Advocating for diabetes awareness and support is essential in raising public understanding, promoting early detection, improving access to care, and enhancing the quality of life for individuals living with diabetes.

Advocacy efforts aim to address the challenges faced by people with diabetes, reduce stigma, and drive policy changes that positively impact diabetes prevention, management, and research. Here are some key aspects of advocating for diabetes awareness and support:

Education and Awareness Campaigns: Advocacy organizations, healthcare providers, and communities conduct educational campaigns to raise awareness about diabetes, its risk factors, and its impact on individuals and society. These campaigns disseminate accurate information about diabetes prevention, early detection, management, and potential complications.

Empowering People with Diabetes: Advocacy initiatives focus on empowering individuals with diabetes to become active participants in their care. This includes providing resources, tools, and support to help them self-manage their condition effectively and make informed decisions about their health.

Policy Advocacy:
Advocacy groups work with policymakers to influence diabetes-related policies at local, national, and international levels. These policies may encompass areas such as healthcare access, insurance coverage, research funding, and workplace accommodations for people with diabetes.

Support Networks and Peer-to-Peer Assistance:
Advocacy organizations often establish support networks and peer-to-peer assistance programs, connecting individuals with diabetes and their families to share experiences, advice, and emotional support.

Advocating for Research Funding:
Advocacy efforts play a crucial role in urging government agencies, private foundations, and industry to invest in diabetes research. Funding for research is

vital to understanding the disease better, finding innovative treatments, and advancing technologies to improve diabetes care.

Reducing Stigma and Discrimination: Advocacy campaigns work to combat stigma and discrimination associated with diabetes. They aim to foster understanding and empathy in society and encourage respectful language and behavior towards individuals with diabetes.

Community Outreach: Advocacy groups engage in community outreach to promote diabetes awareness and offer screenings, educational workshops, and resources. These efforts help identify undiagnosed cases and support early intervention.

World Diabetes Day: World Diabetes Day, observed on November 14th each year, serves as a global platform to raise awareness about diabetes and related issues.

Organizations and individuals around the world participate in activities and events to mark the occasion and advocate for diabetes awareness and support.

Collaboration with Healthcare Providers:
Advocacy groups collaborate with healthcare professionals to enhance diabetes care and support services. They work together to develop comprehensive care plans, educational materials, and resources for individuals with diabetes and their families.

Media and Social Media Engagement:
Leveraging media and social media platforms, advocacy efforts aim to reach a broader audience with diabetes-related information, personal stories, and updates on research and advancements.

By advocating for diabetes awareness and support, individuals and organizations contribute to a collective effort to improve the lives of people with diabetes and work towards a world where diabetes is better understood, well-managed, and prevented. Through collaboration and ongoing advocacy, positive changes can be made to address the challenges posed by diabetes and foster a more supportive and inclusive environment for those affected by the condition.

Conclusion

Diabetes is a complex and chronic condition that affects millions of people worldwide. Understanding the different types of diabetes, their causes, and risk factors is crucial for early detection and effective management. Type 1 diabetes results from an autoimmune response leading to insulin deficiency, while Type 2 diabetes involves insulin resistance and relative insulin deficiency. Gestational diabetes occurs during pregnancy and requires careful monitoring to safeguard both the mother and baby's health.

Insulin plays a vital role in diabetes management by facilitating the uptake of glucose into cells for energy. Proper administration and storage of insulin are essential for maintaining blood sugar levels within a healthy range.

Recognizing common symptoms of diabetes, such as excessive thirst, frequent urination, unexplained weight loss, and fatigue, allows for timely diagnosis and intervention.

Diagnostic tests and procedures, including blood tests and oral glucose tolerance tests, are used to confirm the presence of diabetes and distinguish between Type 1 and Type 2 diabetes.

Building a diabetes management team comprising healthcare professionals, dietitians, educators, and specialists ensures comprehensive and personalized care for individuals with diabetes. A tailored diabetes management plan involves lifestyle adjustments, healthy eating, regular physical activity, and appropriate medications or insulin therapy.

Regular monitoring of blood glucose levels using glucose monitoring devices provides valuable data for adjusting treatment plans and maintaining stable blood sugar levels.

A healthy diet, including carbohydrate counting and considering the glycemic index, is fundamental for diabetes management, while portion control ensures balanced nutrition.

Physical activity offers numerous benefits for diabetics, such as improved insulin sensitivity, cardiovascular health, and overall well-being. Tailoring exercise routines to individual needs and safety considerations is essential for optimal results.

Promising trends in diabetes research, such as closed-loop systems, oral insulin, and precision therapies, hold the potential to revolutionize diabetes care and enhance patient outcomes.

Coping with the emotional aspects of diabetes is equally important, and seeking support, managing stress, and practicing self-compassion are essential components of emotional well-being.

Diabetes management during special circumstances, such as travel and illness, requires careful planning, regular monitoring, and flexibility to maintain optimal blood sugar control.

Advocating for diabetes awareness and support is critical in raising public understanding, driving policy changes, reducing stigma, and empowering individuals with diabetes to manage their condition effectively.

In conclusion, diabetes management is a lifelong journey that requires proactive efforts, a strong support system, and a commitment to maintaining a healthy lifestyle. By staying informed, seeking the support of healthcare professionals, and adopting positive lifestyle adjustments, individuals with diabetes can lead fulfilling lives while effectively managing

their condition and reducing the risk of complications.
Additionally, ongoing research and advancements in diabetes care offer hope for continued improvements in diabetes management and ultimately finding a cure for this prevalent and challenging condition.